Be Real Fit!

A Spiritual Pathway to Victorious Living

By: Loranda Hellen-Thomas, Rph

Kingdom Living Ministries
11601 Shadow Creek Pkwy st.111-193
Pearland, Tx 77584

Virtuous Ink Publishing
PO Box 33
Cibolo, Texas 78108
www.virtuousinkpublishing.com

Printed in the United States of America

ISBN-10: 0988625911
ISBN-13: 978-0-9886259-1-4

The book is dedicated to my loving and faithful husband, Pastor Hermie Thomas, and my devoted children, Judah and Royal Thomas. A special thanks to my mother, Lora Jean Hellen, for teaching and instilling in me love and wisdom.

This book is intended for educational purposes only. It is always important to consult your physician before starting any new diet or exercise plan. All medications and treatments should be continued unless otherwise stated from a primary care physician.
The author of Be Real Fit™ and it's ministry partners are not liable for the misuse of the information presented in this book, nor are we responsible for any loss experienced as a result of the information provided. We are not physicians and are not qualified to give any medical advice.

My *Victorious* Story

As a young girl, I was not raised in the church, yet a belief in God, Jesus, and the Bible was instilled in me. My mom modeled goodness and my dad, a minister, kept us in the Word. Although I was baptized at the young age of 8, I was also raped at the same age. As I became a teenager, I didn't have a personal relationship with Christ, and that caused me to not know how to deal with the physical and emotional pain that comes from such a horrific experience. As a result, I did not know how to handle conflict and often withdrew within myself in order to cope.

As a college student, I witnessed the faith walk of a classmate who later introduced me to Christ. I still did not attend church, but I became very curious. At this time I didn't know that exposure to the truth would make me a mark for the enemy to use my mind as a playground.

I went through disappointment and despair in my relationships which caused me not to trust or believe in the goodness of anyone. I hated my boyfriend, now my husband, although he never gave up on me; even when I decided to move on. He got saved and invited me to church; this opened my eyes and heart to the possibility of forgiveness. The teachings convicted me to the point where I didn't want to do anything but go to church and come home. We were married in 1998, immediately started a family, and enjoyed a wonderful relationship. After seven years, I became numb to my spiritual sensitivity because I began to experience and witness things in the church that were not of God. My innocence was once again shattered and because others were saved and still living like they were in the world, I thought my faith in God would not let anything bad happen to me.

This is where my *victorious* story begins...

The devil moved in on my life and I began to live a very unhealthy lifestyle. In 2006, I left the church and started running with people who were saved but still full of the world. I began to frequent night clubs and thought I might as well *do me* since everyone else was *doing them*. People felt that because I was strong and had my faith I could handle anything, but I was weak and needed deliverance from co-dependence and fear of rejection. THE DEVIL KNEW THIS!

I found myself waking up two years later to an alter ego that had now become my true identity. I did all I could to live up to the person I felt myself becoming; a hypocrite. I remember the Lord called me to preach during these two years and I would cry out, "Who am I? I am so unworthy!" I found myself looking for love that only God could give and I would do almost anything to get it. My husband would pray for me as I would get dress every Friday and head out to dance the night away with so called friends who meant me no good. They were only there for the ride and what I had to offer. I could not see how the enemy used them to get me off course.

In 2008, I said, "Yes I will minister, but Lord you must help me." I started minister's classes and in 2009 entered Fuller Theological Seminary. I was still full of sin and enrolled simply out of obedience. Everyone could see the gifts God had graced me with except for me, but the encouragement from my classmates and Professors put me on the road to self discovery. I begin to blog about my experience and traced my actions back to how I was betrayed and all the hurt and pain that I experienced. I was weak in my faith and put my trust in other people when it should have been in God. The pain of being rejected in the church on several occasions and the pain of others misuse of my trust left me in a state of vulnerability. My relief came only after landing on my face and listening to the voice of God. During this time, the Lord changed my life and my relationship with others in a very profound and unusual way.

Once again I became sensitive to what He said and what He promised in His Word, which led me back to who he had intended me to be. In spite of opposition, I pressed forward and served in ministries and churches that did not and could not accept what I had to offer. It served as a training ground for what I was about to experience.

In 2010, we lost the lifestyle we had come to know; our family business, homes, cars, trucks...we lost everything! Until then, finances were never an issue for us. We lived in gated communities and drove range rovers and Mercedes Benz while our kids were going to the finest private schools in Houston. We lost it all and for two years we lived in an apartment without any income. We tried to cope, but ended up filing bankruptcy. There was so much hardship and pain, I couldn't help but blame myself and my reckless behavior as the cause of my family financial failures. Bad business decisions and the need to have it all caused money to be my master.

In 2012, we moved into another house and received a Word from the Lord that we would both work in government; unbelievably this became true. My husband founded Global Momentum Construction, a commercial construction management company, and I am the Chief Pharmacist for the city of Houston's Health Department. In the mist of it all, God instructed us to start a ministry. We had no money and could have been homeless at any time, but He kept us and honored our faithfulness.

As life progressed, ministry became unbearable and I wanted to give it all up. That's when I had my own *belly of the whale* experience. For three days I stayed in a fetal position crying out, but no one called or asked where I was or even how I was doing. God blocked everyone because it was time, once and for all, that I receive my victory.

This is where my *victorious* story continues...

On the third day, the Lord spoke these words to me:

You are victorious! You've got the victory! I am withholding you and holding you up so you cannot fall or fail. I have called you to be an Apostle; to minister to the world my saving grace. When you get up you are going to have everyone, everything, and the strength you need to complete the task at hand. It is finished.

That very week everyone showed up miraculously to help us fulfill our destiny. I was stunned! Once again, God proved himself to be faithful. I am now living a *victorious* life! The Lord has transformed my mind, body, soul, and spirit, and he has blessed us with every good and perfect thing for His glory. He has His hands on my life, and everything I touch comes forth as pure gold. All that I am and will be belongs to Him. This is the beginning of my second life, another chance to be what I was born to be; a deliverer of a nation.

Today, we have a full time ministry, Kingdom Living Center: Where We Live the Victorious Life. We teach others kingdom principles on victorious living and offer life coaching, bible study, Christian Socials, counseling for rape victors, ministry for children and young adults, and a quarterly Worship service called *The Gathering* designed to minister to the world.

Be Real Fit! A Spiritual Pathway to Victorious Living, is my first book and tells my victorious story in the area of faith, fitness, and fellowship. My second book and stage play, *I Am Victorious,* will be out in the next two years. It depicts the lives of others who are overcoming various challenges through the power of God.

I hope that you will purchase the book for yourself and/or for someone you know and love. It will help to spread the gospel of Jesus and the power of God to overcome the world. Rape, incest, molestation, and the issues associated with these events are very prevalent in the African American community as well as across the nation. We are committed to raising awareness and providing support to those who have had similar experiences.

I have come to realize that God's grace is sufficient and is all I ever really need. It is not perfection that I am after, rather excellence knowing that with God, all things are possible. Charis (Grace and Peace be with you all).

Love,

Loranda "Victorious" Thomas

The Victory Coach
Health and Wellness Coach, Author, and Motivational Speaker

CHAPTER ONE

Let's Get Fit! Mind, Body, Spirit, and Soul

If you are a believer in the Lord Jesus Christ, then you have been born again into the family of God; therefore, you are a child of God. You now hold a position of power, authority, privilege, advantage, and responsibility. This is no small matter to consider.

For years Christians have been living defeated lives in the areas of health and wellness simply because of the choices they make concerning what they eat. Many have been missing out on the great privileges of being a believer; partly because of their lack of knowledge and partly because of Satan's tactics and schemes. So often we find ourselves living and experiencing defeat and destruction when we should be living out the promises of God.

One of these promises found in Isaiah 54:14-15 says, *In righteousness you shall be established; You shall be far from oppression, for you shall not fear; And from terror, for it shall not come near you. Indeed they shall surely assemble, but not because of Me. Whoever assembles against you shall fall for your sake.*

People everywhere are hungry for God and are coming into a spiritual awareness of who they are in Him. They are assembling, but not because of Him. They are filling the void in their lives by replacing the only true and living God with false gods. This results in believers not grabbing hold of the power and provision that God has made in all areas of their lives.

The Apostle John said, "Beloved, I wish above all things that thou may prosper and be in health even as thy soul prospers." Jesus does not only desire your health and prosperity, He died on the cross so that you may prosper and be in good health. Prosperity and health are God's promises available through salvation. It is God's desire that as you come into the knowledge of the spirit of truth, your soul prospers.

It is my sincere hope that through this book, you will discover the power within you to change the way you eat as a lifestyle; if not for your physical health, then at least for your spiritual well being. Acts 10:2 says that those who are devout, fear God and seek Him sincerely. It also says that prayers are answered. If the church is going to experience the promises of God and walk in the fullness of life, this area must be conquered. It is simply a matter of choice between life or death.

Unfortunately, many people do not view food as a false god, a form of idolatry, or something capable of being worshipped. Therefore, they do not consider the sin of overindulgence and gluttony to be a hindrance to their relationship with God. It is a deceitful scheme of Satan to prey on the natural, innate ability of the body to react when hunger is present.

Hunger presents itself in the form of weakness; physical and mental fatigue that creates a desire to eat. The bible says that food is made for the stomach, so it is acceptable as long as one does not allow it to consume them. Consequently, Satan perverts these two truths leading believers to think that since God made everything, then everything can be eaten.

The signs of hunger should be satisfied in the presence of hunger, however, in its absence, erratic and fallible choices are praised as comfort or pleasure leading to the destruction and detriment of one's body and soul. You are in a dangerous place when you break covenant with God by putting something else before Him. Deuteronomy 4:23-24 warns us that God is a jealous God, and will destroy you like a devouring fire if you put anything before Him. Therefore, if you are in an emotional state and choose food to overcome stress and relieve pain and suffering, you are essentially sinning and putting a false god before the living God. God is so perfect and so sufficient that he is jealous, and would destroy you himself if He is not given your affection and loyalty exclusively. He will defend His Word and will not compromise His Spirit.

When you consume unhealthy foods, subconsciously you experience low self-esteem. Your conscious mind then tries to lead you to eat right, but not out of any goodness of your own. It is not your willpower or a battle within your mind. God has a combat for your weakness that He provides only when you put your trust and faith in Jesus, and allow Him to lead you in your choices.

There is only one God-given way to overcome overindulgence, obsessions, and obesity, and that is through the Holy Spirit. According to Luke 2:25, God wants us to not only live a righteous life, but a devout, spirit-filled life which allows us to overcome our sinful desires. Overindulgence of food is a sinful desire; just like smoking, drinking, sex, and gambling. It occupies your mind, time, and money, and causes you to break fellowship and relationship with God. It causes more damage to the spiritual walk than the physical being. We know that the Holy Spirit is more than enough to keep you from drinking, smoking, and indulging in sex. The Holy Spirit is also powerful enough to get rid of the passion and desire to eat unhealthy foods.

Consider how many times you have blamed God for using food as gratification rather than allowing the Holy Spirit to help you overcome the temptation? Also consider how many times you have given in to the temptation of satisfying and addictive foods simply because you believe that it's your vice? How long can you continue to fix yourself up on the outside while the inside is deteriorating at a rapid pace?

More than likely, you are aware that the enemy will put up a fight to prevent you from laying hold of God's promise and provision. Therefore, you must be prepared to *fight the good fight of faith,* knowing that the battle has already been won. There is no substitution for preparedness. We cannot continue to lose hope in the area of health and wellness, pretending the problem does not exist. We can't continue believing that our treasures are stored up in heaven, so we might as well eat and be merry here on earth. Our bodies are the temples of the living God and should be presented Holy and acceptable unto Him, which is our reasonable service.

The body is to be used to bring glory to the Father. It would be an injustice to experience spiritual victory and not conquer the flesh, and control what we put into our own bodies. We have too much ammunition to give our bodies over for destruction by Satan. We have the Name of Jesus, the Blood of Jesus, the Word of God, the spirit of praise, and the Holy Spirit. There is no error in the tearing down of strongholds through the Word of God.

Enough is enough! I am fed up with seeing God's people thinking that they are free, but really they're in bondage. They are slaves to food and don't even realize it. Your Faith in Jesus and what He did on the cross are the keys to your victory. Remember, Ephesians 6:12 says, *our struggle is not against flesh and blood, but against the rulers, against authorities, against the powers of this dark world and against spiritual forces of evil in the heavenly realms*. Therefore it is imperative that we approach this area of our lives spiritually.

We must know, speak, and come into agreement with the Word of God and what it says concerning our lives. Begin to use the Word of God as a weapon in your life. When you pray, it will remove all obstacles that may get in your way. The victory is already yours! Its time to get your inheritance of prosperity and health.

I would be remiss not to tell you that this is a stronghold that is not easy to overcome. My battle with overindulgence came as a result of a lifelong need to give love and be loved in return. I found that food was not going to leave or change; it was predictable and reliable. I could always count on it to do what it was designed to do, and at the time, that was to satisfy my longing to be in a loving, meaningful relationship.

I remember when I was growing up, food was given as a reward and taken away as a form of punishment. This set a pattern that would take me a lifetime to overcome. When I was feeling good I would eat. When I was feeling sad I would eat. My mood dictated whether or not it would be a tasty, crunchy treat or a cream filled desert. I did not realize that what I was doing was setting myself up for failure. There was a deeper battle going on that I could not see: an ongoing battle for my mind, body, and soul. Do you ever notice how your spirit feels based upon when and what you eat? That's your inner man tugging at you, trying to align you with the will of God concerning your emotional wellness. The cycle stops here! Let's make a personal declaration.

Repeat the following **I WILL** statements:

- **I WILL** seek God's wisdom when faced with situations that prompt me to overeat.
- **I WILL** make sure I am not allowing desires to control me.
- **I WILL** confront upsetting situations that I am facing.
- **I WILL** acknowledge that sometimes it's okay to eat *comfort foods* in moderation.
- **I WILL** attempt to understand what triggers my need to overindulge.
- **I WILL** trust God to meet my needs, not food.
- **I WILL** be mindful to keep my needs separate from my wants.

As you begin this journey, there are some things required of you that will help along the way.

1. Make a list of the foods you actually need for the nourishment of your body.
2. Consider how you approach food when in an ideal situation versus a crisis.
3. Ask God to forgive you for looking to food for comfort.
4. Seek God for guidance on how to deal with the urge to overeat.
5. Consider what Jesus did when he was tempted.

6. Choose one thing you can live without that is not beneficial to your health.

There are a few more things that you will need to remember as you take each step on this journey to health and wellness. First, look for God's guidance along the way; do not attempt to overcome this demonic spirit on your own. Don't be surprised when faced with the same temptation; the past does tend to repeat itself, but with God's help you can dodge those tugs toward old behaviors. Look to the scriptures, as Jesus often did, for wisdom and understanding of what it means to live your life in Christ.

You may have to change your environment in order to see lasting change in this area of your life. Throw away anything that you know brings up old memories of your past failures. For instance, take those old size 6 pants that you had from high school and give them to the Goodwill. A size *6* ten years ago is a size *10* now. Also, resist going to the same old restaurants and bars, especially if they tempt you to return to your old nature. Finally, at all costs, avoid relationships that encourage you to look back, and embrace the idea of developing new ones that can propel you into your future.

Points to Ponder

Let's Take Ownership of our own Health

1. Do you think it's God's will for us to be in good health? What steps can you take to bring your will in line with His?

____

____

____

____

2. Consider 1 Thessalonians 5:23, can you identify the process by which God chooses to make you whole?

____

____

____

____

3. According to 2 Corinthians 7:1, who is responsible for the cleansing of our spirit?

____

____

____

____

4. Define *fear*. In what areas of your life do you experience fear?

____

____

____

____

5. Read Ephesians 6:11 and consider who your enemies are?

____

____

____

____

CHAPTER TWO

The Balance of Mind, Body, and Spirit

In Psalm 51:10, David pleaded with God to create in him a clean heart, and renew a right Spirit within him. Knowledge is power, and revealed knowledge is even more powerful. The battle of indulgence can be overcome through the cleansing of the heart and the renewal of the spirit through the mind. When you sin through gluttony, you are replacing God with food, and essentially worshipping another god. You must pray, seek God's will, and ask Him to clean you from within and to fill your heart and mind with new thoughts and desires.

Out of a man's heart comes his thoughts, so if you have given your thoughts over to the power of greed, you can only change that pattern with a clean heart and spirit. This then leads to clean thoughts and desires. There is no need to change your diet if you are not going to change your mind and your relationship with food. Thoughts that are clean, righteous, and pure can eliminate the desire for unclean, wrong, and impure foods. A desire for impure food is a byproduct of impure desires and thoughts. Usually, it's a cover up for fear, weakness, envy, jealousy, or doubt that stem from not knowing and trusting God and His Word.

The moment you overindulge, you give up control of your thoughts and behavior. Without control of your thoughts, it is impossible to achieve any goal or desire. It is only natural to want to appease those desires for impure or unhealthy foods, however, any progress requires great sacrifice. It is a sacrifice because the moment the thought of impure food rises, you are responsible for practicing self-control by casting out the thought, rebuking the demon, and acting wisely. Many people fail in their efforts of weight loss after a short while simply because they give in to their own thoughts. They allow circumstances, people, and the idea of a lifetime of eating healthy to overwhelm them. A lifetime of eating the right foods means a lifetime of righteous thoughts and behavior. God will bless your efforts when you are determined to make the right choices. It is a well-known fact that you will remain in your present state if you give little or no effort.

The first thing that must be done is to get rid of all doubts and fears. They must be absolutely forbidden if you are to successfully gain control over your thoughts. Fears and doubts are caused by repeated failure and paralysis in the spirit. They cause one to relapse into their old lifestyle and cause the disintegration of ones efforts. You must begin to exude positive energy and think positive thoughts on purpose. You can achieve this by thinking highly of yourself. Believe that what you are doing is the only, and best way for you to achieve your goal. Believe that it is your God-given right to be healthy and fit.

As you evolve into a being that thinks positively, you will not only enjoy what you are doing, but you will begin to see meaningful results. Make up your mind today that this is going to be your way of life rather than continue to compromise your health and well being with fad diets. It requires effort to always have healthy, pure, clean, and strong thoughts. However, doing this one thing can build your body, immune system, self-confidence, and overall health. If your mind is consumed with depression, anxiety, unclean thoughts, and negative feelings about yourself or someone else, you cannot have a clean body. No one can put junk into their body and expect to yield grace and beauty. Likewise, no one can put junk into their mind and expect to have joy, peace, happiness, and serenity.

Paul says in Roman 12:1-2 to give your bodies to God, and let it be a living, holy sacrifice; the kind He will accept. When you think of what He has done for you, is this too much to ask? Do not copy the customs and behavior of this world, but let God transform you into a new person by the way you think. Paul is telling us to refuse to conform to the world's behavior and customs, and further lets us know that this is done by deep rooted thoughts planted in our mind. Begin to allow your mind and spirit to lead you, and watch all other gods follow and obey. A renewed heart and spirit not only brings about new, fresh desires and thoughts, it also enables self-control. Philippians 2:13 says, *God is working in you, giving you the desire to obey and the power to do what He wants.* God gives us both the desire, and the power through the Holy Spirit to submit to His control and to allow Him to work in and through us.

To have self-control is to have the power to resist temptation and to allow God to do the rest. We are more than conquerors, and victorious through Christ Jesus. He will take the desire and the need completely away. The moment you make a conscious effort to resist the temptation, it gets stronger. That's the reason that shortly after trying to eat right and make better choices, it's easy to lapse back into worse eating patterns than before. In your human efforts, you lack the patience and endurance to make permanent changes. Time and time again you start a diet or weight loss plan, and fail to complete even one week successfully. This is the reason Paul says to put no confidence in your human effort.

Will power never produces lasting results. The temptation that the devil uses regarding eating is too strong to overcome with mere will power. However, you do have the power to resist. How do you resist a temptation that's natural, desirable, and beneficial when used properly? I'm glad you asked!

First, realize that being tempted is not a sin. I am going to say it again, ***being tempted is not a sin***. In other words, unless the gallon of ice cream is eaten after the crisis, you have not sinned. Do not let the enemy of your mind make you think that just because you thought it, you might as well do it; that is a lie from the pits of hell. When you're tempted, simply pray for the strength to resist rather than give in to the temptation. In some instances you must literally run, especially in the face of persistent temptation. This is the only solution if you want the victory. Finally, when confronted with that which you know is not good for your health, speak out against it and do not be apologetic about it. Once Satan is resisted, rebuke all of the tactics that he used to get you to indulge. Whether it's doubt, discouragement, disappointment, diversion, defeat, or delay, call it out. Rebuke it and allow the Holy Spirit to lead you into greater awareness of your ability to make better choices for your health.

Food, as all things are, is a gift from God and should be enjoyed. It should not be used for comfort or to relieve pain, but for proper nourishment, to preserve ones health, and give energy to serve God. Food should not be used as a reward for being good or to overcome boredom or loneliness. As Paul states in Titus 1:16, *everything is pure to those whose hearts are pure. Nothing is pure to those who are corrupt and unbelieving because their minds and conscious are defiled.* Such people claim to know God, but they deny Him in the way they live. They are despicable and disobedient, not worthy of doing anything. Those who are pure have Christ as their center and are in control of their lives. They love the things that are pure and good; even food. As you begin to practice this way of living in this area, you will soon find the good in all things as you allow God to fill your hearts and minds.

Lying and deceiving spirits who are greedy for money have turned many Christians from what they know and believe is right and true when it comes to their own health. This book is written for Christians, even if they reject, disbelieve, and disobey God in this area. Religious and familial traditions play a vital role in the customs and behaviors of the average Christian. Paul cautions us in 1 Timothy 4:16 to keep a close watch on yourself and your teachings. The scripture says that if you stay true to what is right, God will save you and those who hear you.

Wrong beliefs and teachings can lead people into sin, and cause many to follow a path of unrighteousness because they do not see the necessity of being both spiritually and physically fit. Always be weary of anyone who says you can lose weight simply by taking a pill or following a diet without behavioral modification. There is no magic potion or one type of pill, vitamin, or food that is the key to a healthy lifestyle.

On the other hand, do not be deceived by false teachings that say all you need for good health is in the foods that we eat. Anyone who exerts themselves, whether it's in the home or at work, needs additional vitamins and nutrients to supplement their food intake and recharge their bodies. Although our faith and belief in God can sustain us through anything, our physical bodies are subject to decay and disease. No man can live a long, pain-free life without the proper balance of nutrients and vitamins.

It is my mission to dispel the lie that we do not have to take care of ourselves because of our faith in God. After God saw me through a personal struggle with food, I know that victory does not come through inactive faith. It takes the right combination of vitamins, nutrients, herbs, and food to fuel your body and to prevent it from craving fats and sweets. In order for the body to expel and function at its peak, it must be supplied with what it needs to reach its potential.

A lot of the despair we feel is a result of the types of food we eat. Certain foods such as sugar, wheat, diary, and white flour are the culprit for many illnesses that result in chemical and hormonal imbalances. What you are is directly linked to what you eat, but that does not mean *you are what you eat*. What it means is that you are the sum total of what you eat, think, breathe, and most of all, what you believe. Do not believe the enemy that says you are not good enough because you struggle in this area. Harmony in the mind, body, and spirit requires a perfect balance of the right thoughts, emotions, feelings, desires, nutrients, and movement. All of this can be controlled through the spirit, but it requires our active participation. The more we are in tune with our mind and body, the less resistant we become to change. Yes, you will experience withdrawal symptoms such as fatigue, boredom, and complacency similar to those seen with drugs and alcohol, but the results will be phenomenal! You will look better, feel better, and gain a new sense of purpose when you make better food choices.

The spirit is able to cure and heal any disease and deliver you from any addiction. God is our creator and sustainer, and all power is in His hands. However, our physical bodies must be in the state that God created it to be in to experience the power of health and healing promised to the descendants of Abraham. In other words, it's hard to receive the blessings of the Father if we are not in the proper state to receive Him. Contrary to what many Christians believe, God works best with what we have. That should motivate us to take care of our bodies and minds since they are the only ones we have.

Disease is caused when our bodies simply stop working properly. When we are not living a life in harmony with God, self, and others our hypothalamus takes emotions like fear, anxiety, anger, etc., and translates them into chemical messages that cause every organ in our body to start over or under producing hormones and neurotransmitters. We can handle this over or under production for a short period of time, but when it happens chronically, our body becomes damaged which causes disease.

Another way that we develop disease is when we harbor anger or bitterness against one another. It does not affect the other person, but us. When fear and anxiety rule our lives, it shows that we do not trust God, and that is hypocritical. Living a life of hypocrisy is a sin and opens up the door to all sorts of other demonic forces. Many diseases are spiritual in nature, and must be dealt with on a spiritual level. We cannot expect to be blessed and in good health when we are knowingly operating in sin. We not only have to repent of our sins and change, but we must also deal with the spiritual forces that are behind our physical issues. God cannot anoint that which he does not bless, and healing cannot take place where there is no anointing. His anointing falls in the areas he has blessed, gifted, or given revelation in. Psalm 68:19 says, *Blessed be the Lord, who daily loadeth us with benefits, even the God of our salvation.*

Dealing with our sin and overcoming hypocrisy does not come without great effort, but the result is astronomical! God anoints those who use their natural, God-given ability to bring about His divine purpose. God shows us in His word that when he calls us for His purpose, he uses the very skills he has already given; he does not create new ones. Take the disciple Matthew for example. When he decided to follow Jesus, he was given a new life. He was a despised tax collector, but God gave him a new purpose for that skill and made him a record keeper. He was a keen observer and recorded everything he saw.

We are God's workmanship and a work in progress. What He gave to us, He gave long before we came to realize and responded to it. You have what it takes to rebuild the body you have, God is not going to give you a new one. However, He can give you a new life and anoint the body you have to wellness! What you tried in the past does not amount to the knowledge you are about to gain, and knowledge is the key to success. Once you unleash the power of what you learn, no one will be able to take it from you. You will then be empowered to overcome the sin of overindulgence and help others to do the same. Let go of the excuse that you are too old, too fat, too tired, and too busy. Grab hold of the promise of the Father to supply all your needs according to His riches that are in Christ Jesus.

The balance of the mind, body, spirit, and soul is so intricately connected that it can make you spiritually estranged and mentally distressed if they are not in harmony. I remember a time when my life was extremely scattered and utterly out of control, and for the longest time I did not understand why. I had to revisit a life altering situation in order to understand what had gotten me to this point of insanity.

At the age of eight, I was raped by a complete stranger who took my innocence and robbed me of my purity. Being violated through sexual abuse can cause your entire life to become discombobulated. To make matters worse, I was told and believed that it was my fault. Believing this lie caused me to be victimized all over again. This horrific childhood experience opened the door to a life long battle with an identity crisis and an internal conflict that I suppressed for many years. I would cling to those who told me they loved me, and would do anything to keep them around.

It would send me into an emotional crisis whenever a friendship or love relationship ended. I would always think it was my fault, and as a result I was constantly in unhealthy relationships that would prove to be detrimental to my mental and emotional wellness. I often found myself in compromising situations and could not recognize what caused me to be this way.

I do not blame anyone else because I realize the problem was not with them but with me. I put my trust in people to satisfy certain areas of my life when I should have only trusted in God. Only God can love you unconditionally. Only He is worthy of the trust and admiration that I was putting in people. It's okay to acknowledge those great character traits found in others, but to rely on them for your mental and spiritual well-being is idolatry.

I repeatedly received a false pretense of love that was based upon what I can give rather than pure agape love. Is it possible? Does it really exist? Can men and women really have loving, fulfilling relationships and not cross those boundaries? Can females truly love each other, without being jealous or stabbing each other in the back? Can a person really love with the love of God in a way that brings health and healing, or does this only exist in heaven?

I came to realize that these types of healthy relationships are not only possible, but a *reality*! I trusted people to a fault, but it caused me to open up to God and pray in a way I never had before. It brought me to a place of pain that made me think, *how did I get here* and *how can I get pass this place*?

At my breaking point, God spoke these words to me, "Mortify therefore your members which are upon the earth; fornication, uncleanness, inordinate affection, evil concupiscence, and covetousness, which is idolatry" (Colossians 3:5). These words proved to be life changing, and served as the key that unlocked my deliverance and set me free.

Let's examine the text. Read Colossians 3:5 once more and find yourself in it. What does it say to you? Are you out of balance because of the things you have done in your body? Have these things affected your mind? Well, here is the good news; you can be set free!

Jesus says, "If the Son makes you free you should be free indeed" (John 8:36). You have been set free from sin and have become a slave to righteousness (Romans 6:18). You are no longer a slave you are free, but your freedom is not an excuse to do evil. You are free to live as God's slave (1 Peter 2:16). Stand fast therefore in the liberty by which Christ has made you free, and do not be entangled again with a yoke of bondage (Galatians 5:1). Having been set free from sin and becoming a slave of God, you have your fruit to holiness, and in the end everlasting life (Romans 6:22). Once you were under God's curse, doomed forever for you sins (Ephesians 2:1), but now you are aware and will not let your liberty become a stumbling block to those who are weak. (1 Corinthians 8:9).

I found out that what I thought was freedom was really bondage. My motto was, *do anything I want, anytime, and anywhere.* You only live once right? ***Wrong***! What you do has an impact on the lives of others. Your freedom comes with responsibility.

Paul speaks about a freedom that comes from being in a relationship with Christ; that's the only true freedom. God restored my mind, body, spirit, soul, and marriage. Every covetous spirit that even entered into my mind had to flee. The spirit of inordinate affection that once had me bound loosed its hold once I grabbed a new freedom found only in Christ. If you want to experience true freedom, begin to consider what is right in *every* situation. Show concern and be responsible for others by the way you behave around them. Choose your words and actions carefully, knowing that someone is watching you. That should motivate you to want to live responsibly.

I never had a clear understanding of what Romans 6:18 meant when it refers to being a *slave to righteousness*. I now know that it means that we must have appropriate boundaries and not let anyone cause us to lower our standards. Remember, freedom means something different to you than it does to someone else.

Since I have been set free, I refuse to allow anyone to use me or abuse my kind heart for his or her gain. I now respect others by showing restraint in my thoughts, words, and actions. In all you do, seek to live according to Jesus' principle of love.

In the early church, Paul sought out and recommended people of good reputations for key roles in the ministry. Know that when you seek to be like Jesus, you will earn a good reputation. Do not worry about what other people think or feel about you. If God has brought you out of a situation that you know only He could; tell somebody, and watch God use it for your good! Begin to thank God for forgiving you of your sins. Seek his guidance on forgiving those who intentionally used and misguided you into harm's way.

It may be that the people who damaged you didn't do it intentionally. It's possible that they were damaged and did only what they knew to do. People who have been hurt, hurt others in return. When someone comes to remind you of your past, dismiss him or her and carry on. You have come too far in your faith walk to turn back now. God has a way of caring for and preserving us until we can see our way through. You are no longer a victim of your circumstances or your past. You are a ***victor***! Live in the freedom of your spirit. Say it loud, ***I am victorious in Christ Jesus!***

Repeat these **I WILL** statements:

1. **I WILL** remember that the greatest source of love comes from God.
2. **I WILL** enjoy life knowing that I am created in God's image and His likeness.
3. **I WILL** feel good about myself despite what I have been through.
4. **I WILL** remember that God loves *who I am* regardless of *what I do.*
5. **I WILL** remain free and not revert back to my old sins.
6. **I WILL** count on God's Spirit to help me maintain my purity and dignity during life's challenging times.
7. **I WILL** remember that He who has begun a good work in me will continue his work until it is finally finished in that day when Christ Jesus comes back again (Philippians 1:6).
8. **I WILL** not let my heart condemn me, because my confidence is in God (1 John 3:21).

Know that God's love for you is beyond compare. He loves us so much that He sent His son just to die for you and me. Be thankful that God loved you enough to give you a new chance to know Him in a new way. If I hadn't been through the wilderness and the valley, I would not be having the Canaan and Mountaintop experience that I am having now. His love is personal, and no one can replace or come close to it. You must realize that His love is eternal and accept that it's always near because it comes from a different place.

This week, try to find ways to express your gratitude for God's love. For example, you could go to someone who has wronged you and offer them forgiveness, or you could simply say hello to a stranger. Whatever you choose, make up your mind that you are going to show someone the everlasting love and kindness that God has so graciously bestowed upon you. Finally, remember that *hope does not disappoint, because the love of God has been poured out into our hearts by the Holy Spirit who was given to us* (Romans 5:5). There is life after the pain. ***Live it***!

Points to Ponder

Let's find a healthy Balance

1. Consider how disease enters the body? How can you change the course of your life and decrease the chance of developing disease?

2. The ministry of reconciliation is the only way we can be free from disease (Read 2 Corinthians 5:18-21). What does this mean to you? How can the ministry of reconciliation affect your health?

3. What can you do today to be healed from disease and achieve wellness?

CHAPTER THREE

Shake, Rattle, and Role

Many people agree with experts that exercise is important and is needed to be healthy, vibrant, and physically fit. Even the Christian Community is finally beginning to accept the fact that exercise is a necessity, and pushing back from the table is a gift to be desired. I experience great joy when I find new studies that support the idea that it's not the quantity of exercise, but the quality and type of exercise that makes the difference. It's a relief to know that a more moderate approach is best when it comes to healthy fat loss.

People all over the world are having conversations about lowering their fat, sugar, and salt intake. They can do this by eating less meat, dairy, and processed foods and eating more complex carbohydrates and fiber such as whole grains, fresh fruits, and vegetables. In addition, many are incorporating a more active lifestyle by participating in activities such as dancing, stretching, and walking verses strenuous hours of cardio at the gym. Even with these efforts, many people fall short of their goal of having a healthy weight and lifestyle.

The low carb, high-protein craze has left the world starving for a more sensible approach to fast and permanent changes in their weight. Many believe that most diseases require medical intervention in addition to a lifestyle change. However, there is evidence that simple changes can have astonishing results and do not require medical intervention at all. I am in no way advocating or supporting the idea that medical doctors are not necessary. I am simply supporting the idea that disease prevention is possible and capable of being achieved prior to a person reaching a diseased state that requires medical intervention.

There is no quick or easy way to lose fat without sacrifice. For instance, one way to achieve fat loss is to eliminate all flour, starch, and sugary products including bread, pastas, and pastries for a certain period of time. This allows your body's biological clock to resume working properly.

For ten years I have been developing a program that has helped thousands of people lose unwanted weight and gain a healthier lifestyle by changing their eating patterns. Once a person has reach a healthy weight using this program, they are able to adapt a more permanent lifestyle that includes low sugar fruits, healthy starches, less protein from meat, eggs and beans in moderation, and a variety of delicious, mouth-watering vegetables!

The fear of making such changes is as harmful as the fear of death.

Parting ways with your old lifestyle is never an easy task, but your body will thank you for it. You are worth the effort, even if you never reach your final goal. Never give up on the one thing that's sure to make your life better, and that is making healthier choices. Here are a few simple steps that contribute to a healthy lifestyle.

- Keep it very simple; too much variety makes for too much work.
- Eat meals slowly and only take in foods that are beneficial for your well-being.
- Purchase a good plant based cookbook.
- Begin a family tradition of cooking meals that contain more vegetables and less meat and fats.

The program founded by Dr. John A. McDougall is based on common starches such as oatmeal, rice, corn, whole-grain breads, bagels, pastas, white potatoes, sweet potatoes, brown rice, beans, and squash. Fresh and frozen fruits and vegetables are added to theses staples in the McDougall Program. In addition, low-fat soy or rice milk is used instead of daIry and eggs. This way of eating helps to eliminate many ailments caused by the Western diet and overindulgence.

I personally follow an intermittent-fasting type of diet on most days with two days of normal meals. This means that I eat the majority of my calories in the evening and in one sitting. I drink a protein shake or eat a protein bar with super greens in the morning, and green vegetables and salads as I desire during the day. In the evening, I eat a high starch vegetarian meal or a meal made up of protein and vegetables. I call this *Be Slim*, and it is a simple approach to healthy fat-loss.

I followed a strict vegetarian diet for many years and found it helpful in maintaining my health and weight as long as I incorporated high intensity exercises. However, as I got older, I realized that to maintain muscle you have to feed them protein. Therefore to maintain my ideal weight, I must be careful how I incorporate starches into my diet. Portion control is paramount as well as exercises that use my own body. I used PraiseMoves™ developed by Laurette Willis in conjunction with a program that I developed called **Rhema**-*cises* and I found them to be the key to stabilizing my weight. I also incorporate a plant and starch based diet with a moderate amount of lean meats, and eliminated the meat based diets found in Western cultures. These diets are also typically high in fat, cholesterol, and sugar

A more sensible approach is easier to maintain if it is a gradual transition. Start with these simple steps.

- Add vegetables to your meals.
- Start eliminating obviously unhealthy foods such as processed and fried food.
- Start preparing meals at home using fresh produce and whole grains.
- Use meat as a side dish rather than the main course.
- Make good starches the staple of your diet.
- Eliminate meat or use it as a treat a couple of days a week.

Family traditions are important, but do not let the spirit of familiarity cause you to ruin your hard fought efforts to make permanent lifestyle changes. You should frequently read about ways to incorporate vegetables into your favorite recipes, and plan your days so that you can have the things you absolutely love like chocolate or ice cream. Do not wait until you are at a point where you have to decide what you will allow into your body. Also, do not be too hard on yourself and make allowances for mishaps.

The disciples gained spiritual awareness through evolution. They did not come to the point where they knew Jesus and His purpose overnight. It was a gradual process; one that took patience and perseverance, so don't give up just because you do not see your desired results immediately. Jesus didn't give up on the disciples when their hearts were hardened due to unbelief. He simply used every opportunity to get them to see from the perspective that He empowered them to see from. Eventually, they came to the place where they realized the power they had through faith in Christ. That is the same thing that will happen to you.

Once you give up control of yourself to God and allow Him to guide you in your efforts, He will lead you into the truth that you have the power to overcome. The devil has been dethroned, and Christ has been enthroned; you only have to realize it. Do not get sidetracked by what you see as the crowd who was following Jesus did. This limits your access to what Christ can reveal to you. Let go, and let God have His way concerning your food choices. He has been waiting on you to give Him this area of your life just as you have given up control in other areas. There is no stopping a yielded vessel. Years and years of neglecting your body can wreak havoc on your health, but it can all be reversed in a matter of months. Start today and give yourself 100 days to be well again!

Playing it safe has gotten you in the predicament you are in right now. Step out of your comfort zone and believe that you have the victory. Determination plus the right situation coupled with education produces results. It is God's plan for your life that you prosper and be in good health, even as your soul prospers. Take the back seat and humble yourself before the Lord, then watch Him exalt you in due season. Discover this *fit* you, and then lead your family and friends by example.

You have an assignment from the Lord to do, and you are obligated to be at your best when doing it. We are all called to live a more active lifestyle; one in which we do a little more and walk a little farther. We are stewards over our bodies and will be required to give an account of how we use it. Ask yourself these questions:

- As a representative of Christ, do you represent the Kingdom with excellence?
- When people see you, do they see the beauty and radiance on the outside that matches the love and greatness on the inside?
- Will someone want to know Jesus simply by the way they view your outside appearance?

You never know who is watching you, and you never have a second chance to make a first impression. Shake, rattle, and roll your body until the enemy falls under your feet. It doesn't matter what it is, just start your program by doing something. Do not hesitate or procrastinate. Don't let another day go by wishing you could look like anything or anyone other than your beautiful self.

Discover the power of trusting that God is in control of your life by leaning not to your own understanding, and by acknowledging Him in all your ways. You are secure enough in yourself to leap out on faith and take a breath of fresh air during a morning walk. Unleash your dog and run beside him in the evening before dinner. Turn off the television, turn on the radio, and dance the night away. Have family time on bikes after the time spent at the dinner table. Learn a new DVD like PraiseMoves™, and stretch and move your body into shape. You have nothing to lose except stress, fat, and an old mindset.

Perhaps your faith has been an excuse for you not to exercise, but today you are going to make moving your body as important as moving mountains. Make praising and dancing your morning worship, and enjoy **Rhema**-*cises*, which is tailor-made from the Word of God just for you. Intertwined into all of that, what you are called to do is to move your body into its destiny!

For many years I lived under the ostriches that exercise is of the devil. How did I get there? Well, for many years prior to that I ate nothing but healthy food and exercise two to three times a day! I was extremely fit and was proud of it. I did not understand how people could be fat and out of shape when there was something that could be done about it. That was until I went from 150 pounds to 220 pounds following two pregnancies in two years. I never had a weight problem or a problem with food before, and I did not know how to cope with the changes in my body and my hormones.

I tried everything to get back into shape, and literally spent hundreds of thousands of dollars trying to get back into my high school and college clothes. Nothing worked, until I discovered the HCG diet. I am not advocating HCG here and I no longer recommend it to my clients, but that diet is what restored my hypothalamus and hormones back to their proper state.

After various failed weight loss business ventures, I finally found what would become the only way to successfully lose fat and maintain muscle. I opened a clinic that helped many people lose weight and regain their health. Because of challenging Texas regulations, I have since closed the clinic, but I've set out on a mission to get the same results without the necessary doctors, nurses, or needles.

In 2010, I begin to test a program called *Be Slim* that for a certain amount of time followed the same diet of protein, vegetables, and low sugar fruit. It was followed by a healthy eating plan that included beans, eggs, and whole grains. It was the best thing I had ever done!

I maintained the weight loss for more than a year until I experienced the horrific loss of a thriving business that was my families sole income. We could have been homeless had it not been for God. Once the Lord blessed me with another job and my husband with another business, I was ready to get back into shape. I thought I would be able to just cut back, but that didn't happen. I remember thinking, *wow something is different.* I realized that I was 39 and couldn't just cut back anymore and see significant weight loss.

I begin to work out with a trainer and became very discouraged and disinterested in working that hard for mediocre results. I thought about HCG, but immediately thought, *no way, I am not going there.* I had just lost weight without it and was positive that I could do it again. I begin the *Be Slim* plan and set out to do what I did a year ago, before my relapse.

I designed *Be Slim* meals and work outs that took just 10 minutes in the morning and evening. I also added 20 minutes of walking and jogging a few days a week. I called the exercises **Rhema**-*cises* because every morning I would do them to inspirational music and accompany it with a scripture for the day. These exercises were created just for me.

I found myself looking forward to getting up and sharing this time in the Lord with my husband. More than that, I notice that my body begin to change. I begin to see incredible results, just as I did before and knew I wanted to share them with the world. With that, I birthed a seven week wellness lifestyle designed to get you fit, healthy, and living your dreams! I made up my mind that I was going to finish this book by the beginning of 2013. Once again, I wanted to do something that I loved to do.

I am a Pharmacist, a licensed and ordained minster, as well as a health and wellness coach. I will graduate from seminary school soon, and I'm studying to be a Health and Faith Ambassador. I'm armed and ready to serve those who want to lose weight and gain health and wellness naturally.

Right now, begin to confess and profess, "This is my time and my year. I am going to do all I can to to do my level best, and get in the best possible shape for me. The rest I am going to leave up to God to complete what He has begun unto perfection upon His return."

Points to Ponder

Let's get moving

1. In your own words, explain PraiseMoves™ and **Rhema**-*cises* and what these exercises can do to improve your health?

____

____

____

____

2. In addition to PraiseMoves™ and **Rhema**-*cises*, how can you incorporate more activities into your life?

____

____

____

____

3. What time of day and how often can you commit to exercise?

____

____

- *Keep in mind that to lose fat and see significant results, you should exercise daily for at least 100 days.*

CHAPTER FOUR

The Nerve of You

There is a misconception in the church that once you are saved, you are free from all struggles, pain, disappointment, and heartaches. Many are led to believe that frequent visitation to the House of the Lord will somehow ease the problems of everyday life. A great many Christians are confused because they are experiencing defeat in their life in an area that is socially accepted. Great people have had mental instabilities making it *normal* to be agitated, irritated, and full of fear and anxiety, even though we have received all that we need pertaining to life and godliness.

Common sense tells us to seek medical intervention when we're feeling down and out rather than seeking the only true source of joy and comfort. The condition of the nerves commonly referred to as *anxiety* shows up for many different reasons and in many different aspects of the life of the believer. It simply shows that the love of God has not been perfected, and that there is still a great deal of self-reliance at the heart of the matter.

You can overcome this condition by making up your mind and deciding in your heart that you have no power to control the situation. Giving up the need to be in control frees you to live a life of servitude and gratitude. It opens the door to all other aspects of your life under the authority of Christ. Let's first define where these nervous conditions originate from.

Nervousness, anxiety, depression, compulsiveness, possessiveness, obsessions, low self-esteem, emotional, irrational, and relational issues all stem from one common source; a false reality of one's identity. Identity crisis is the culprit of all conditions of the nerves. Being out of touch with one's true feelings and one's true sense of self leads to emotional and relational disorders. To overcome overindulgence, self-indulgence must first be dealt with. In other words, a wake up call into reality is essential if you are going to rid yourself of the persistent pains of being out of touch with who you really are.

Just as spiritual decisions cannot be made in the mist of anxiety and fear, rational decisions concerning your health and well-being cannot be made in the presence of anxiety and fear. Knowledge of your emotions and true desires is the first step to freeing your nerves and experiencing the fullness of life. When decisions are made out of your true desires rather than fear, rarely is there any frustration or regrets. Self-defeating actions, behaviors and thoughts, negligence of proper nourishment of the mind, body, and spirit, lack of self-control, and the fear of intimacy and love all confine us to ourselves, causing the believer to live in a box.

Life should not be lived in constant fear, or constrained by constant thoughts of inhibition. Life should be lived to the fullest in the liberty and freedom offered only through Christ. Emotional, behavioral, and relational problems can be extremely painful and disruptive to the natural flow of one's life. The mind, which houses our psyche, has many functions, but nothing compares to its main function which is survival.

We are in a constant fight for survival. We all adapt to life and the circumstances surrounding it in different ways. The mind working to adapt to anxiety is no different from a person who does what is necessary to gather food to eat. Survival mode is the way we respond when we try to adapt to danger. This is a false reality. When we choose not to deal with reality, we find ourselves in a state of constant struggle through what is commonly called a defense mechanisms.

Defense mechanisms are the reactions to the situations we face with a distorted reality or even a lie. In other words, it's a state of denial to protect against harm. Drinking, sex, drugs, and many other defenses simply bury the true feelings and suppress the truth of the situation. Unless we look beyond our present state, the end result is always the believer living life in a box and being constrained in their own little world. It's time to get out of the box!

The truth of the matter is that Christ is your reality! This truth on an intellectual level does not free us to live the life God has planned for us. There must be a deeper, more profound experience to solidify your faith in Christ and free your mind from the struggles of holding on to a false reality. Hope in Christ and His purpose is what keeps us in tune with our inner-self. Our relationship with ourselves is the problem, not our relationship with Christ. He is not flawed, we are. The moment we realize this truth is the moment we will be on our way to restoration, recovery, and ultimately reality.

Our past experiences and how we view them in terms of negativity or positivity plays a role in how we accept Christ into our lives at the core and allow Him to change us. This is no easy task. A defense response that you have used for your entire life as a coping mechanism often becomes a way of life that works only for you. This can hinder your relationship with Christ and others.

The unconscious mind is fully engaged and is trying to hold on to the old way of life in an effort to keep you *safe* from harm. This is a trick of the devil. Exposure allows for the unconscious mind to be used to lead one into a glorious Christ filled life as your reality. Expose your defense mechanism and set your mind free. Bring your unconscious mind onto the scene and make it face your new reality. Consider these questions:

- What have you used to cope with your situation and maintain your self-image?
- How has your superego gotten you to act in a way that is socially acceptable?
- What has been subconsciously causing you to go against your inner feelings, desires, and spirit?
- What has happened in your childhood to drive you to a place where you feel you have to protect who you are and what you stand for?

Let down the walls of division hindering you from fully embracing your new life in Christ. Feelings of guilt, embarrassment, and shame that accompany anxiety are the defenses that the subconscious uses to lessen the feel of the pain that is feared. It is not real; it's a false reality. Christ is the reality you live in now, and He has come to set the captives free. Allow your identity to reside in Christ alone. There is no other way to overcome this form of oppression then to surrender your will to His, and allow him to heal you from the inside out.

Romans 12:2 says, *Do not conform any longer to the pattern of this world, but be transformed by the renewing of your mind.* It is the Holy Spirit that shapes and conforms; all we have to do is cooperate and bring Christ into our lives as we submit to Him. If you want to be pleasing to God and approved by men, make every effort to do what leads to peace and mutual edification (Romans 14:17-19). We cannot obtain that which is Spiritual by human effort (Galatians 3:3). We must mutually fix our eyes on Jesus, the author and perfecter of our faith (Hebrews 12:2).

I remember when God laid upon my heart the need to deal with some deep-rooted personal issues. I never thought that I could be delivered from them because it was a socially accepted and normal issue for many. How many people are quietly suffering from low-grade depression, loss of control over their life, a loss of spiritual sensitivity, and the loss of a connection with others?

Many people are busy, but extremely bored and find anything to use as a substitute for their lack of restfulness and satisfaction. This comes across as normal because it is said to be just a bad habit like impulsive shopping, unhealthy eating and drinking habits, and a lack of control over personal temptations. It was the Word of God that allowed me to see that these thing are not normal, and that a deep spiritual transformation from within needed to take place.

I allowed God to take me through a period of personal purification. I had to confess my sins and ask for forgiveness, then commit to a daily lifestyle of being renewed through prayer and meditation on His Word. Months and weeks went by, and all I was allowed to do was worship and thank Him. I celebrated life in order to regain sensitivity to the spirit. The more I sought God, the more different I seemed to be compared to others. I resolved that I wouldn't fight the process, and the journey began.

The good thing is that none of us have arrived at the finish line. I am still on the journey, but the decision to follow after the things of God was the best decision I have made in my entire life. Endurance became my middle name, and long suffering my first and last. As I allowed the Spirit of God to shape my character to be more like Christ's character, the more I found myself in a place where my faith was being tried to see if I truly loved the Lord God with all my heart, soul, and strength. The hurts, unfairness, and undermining seemed to get worse, yet the stretching and shaping impacted the core of my soul, and made me into the person I am today. Yielded, willing, obedient, and trusting in the presence of God and the promise that He is with me. This has made me an available vessel to be used by God for the redemption of people.

I have learned to place the weightier matters before the Lord and allow Him to instruct me on how I am to respond. This has given me a new freedom and opened up my mind to the possibilities of a fresh outlook on things that would usually cause me to stumble and fall.

I want to encourage you to make anxiety work in your favor by doing the following:

- Identify those things you have no power to change; acknowledge that you are powerless to change them and move on.
- Prioritize your life and look to reduce your *to-do* list, responsibilities, and expectations.

- Ask for help. Seek a friend, a coach, or someone else who can help you identify what is warranted to be a worry and what is not, then let go and enjoy your life.
- Do not let worry cause you to get weary in well doing. Worry less and trust God more.

I have attempted to reveal the truth concerning your health and well-being from a very spiritual and personal perspective. This work is not exhaustive, but it is designed to get you to a state of self-awareness and to heal yourself with your choices. No one knows everything, but I can tell you that after helping thousands of people achieve their weight loss goals and maintain a healthy weight for the last ten years, the whole person has to be addressed. There is no stopping someone who is aware of the situation they are in. It allows you the opportunity to make an informed decision.

It is my sincere hope today that you make a decision to first, start living your life for Christ and not for yourself. Next, allow the Lord to lead you into making better decisions concerning your health and mental wellness. Finally, I hope that if you are not able to do any of this on your own you will seek professional help.

Every good coach has a coach, and I am no exception. It takes a multitude of counsel to finally reach your goal in this arena. Seek help while you can and live the best life you can through Christ Jesus who strengthens you!

Points to Ponder

Let's be healed in our Mind

1. Read Romans 12:2 and consider how your mind is renewed or cleansed. How can this benefit your emotional well-being?

____

____

____

____

2. According to John 8:32, you shall know the truth and the truth shall make you free. What is your truth?

____

____

____

____

3. Read 2 Corinthians 10:5. What does it mean for you to cast down imaginations and bring into captivity every thought to the obedience of Christ?

____

CHAPTER FIVE

Be Real Faith: Faith not Fear

In order for healing to take place, the ministry of reconciliation in the heart on all levels must first take place. *There is no fear in love, but perfect love casts out fear because fear has torment. He that has fear is not made perfect in love* (1 John 4:18). Love is the main factor in being on the pathway to wellness. There is absolutely no fear in love, so why are we constantly living our lives bound by fear? Self-hatred, guilt, shame, and resentment give way to the spiritual manifestation of fear. This fear allows the enemy an opportunity to make physical manifestation through our natural fight or flight response. This causes adrenaline to be released in the body and hormones to become imbalanced leading to a disconnection between the mind, body, spirit, and soul.

The only way to overcome fear is to once again come into right standing and fellowship with God the Father, The Holy Sprit, and The Son. This is essentially what *Be Real Faith* is about; getting back to the state in our mind that we are responsive and reactive only to the voice of God, not our own or that of others. This is true healing. Are you ready for it? Are you ready to be free to love God like you did when you first believed? You have suffered the consequences of your wrong choices and behaviors long enough. Now is the time to make God your one and only choice. Fear of rejection, fear of man, fear of failure, and fear of abandonment have ruled your life long enough. It's time for you to be loved perfectly. Perfect love cast out *all* fear.

Lack of *real* faith is a real problem in the church. If we take an honest look at ourselves and survey how we have responded to life events, we will realize that our faith has been tainted with fear and that is a sin. Whatever is not faith is sin, therefore Satan wishes to demolish your faith and cause you to live in a constant state of fear. *But without faith it is impossible to please God* (Hebrews 11:6). Satan knows we have not been loved properly and that is a weakness, especially for women. We struggle so much in the area of love, simply because we can handle it. *There are no temptations taken you but such as is common to man: but God is faithful, who will not suffer you to be tempted above ye are able; but will with the temptation also make a way of escape, that ye may be able to bear it* (1 Corinthians 10:13).

You might as well stop asking God to deliver you from fear. He wants you to get to the root of the problem and defeat the temptation that tries to get you out of fellowship with Him and into fellowshipping with the devil. There you have it. The devil is after you in this area because he knows you have the power and ability to overcome him. The bible says, *Blessed is the man who endureth temptation: for when he is tried he shall receive the crown of life which the Lord hath promised to them that love him* (James 1:12).

You may be asking, "What if I do not have faith?" I'm glad you asked. The bible says that *faith comes by hearing and hearing by the Word of God* (Romans 10:17). Therefore, in order to get faith, one must be taught the Word of God. In Luke 18:8, the bible asks if the Son of Man will find real faith on earth when He comes? The church is teaching that all a person has to do is to believe on Jesus Christ, yet what's being produced is a weak, fake faith that the book of James calls dead.

Real, living faith produced by having a true heartfelt belief in God causes one to be convicted into a faith that produces righteousness. So the *Be Real* philosophy answers the question, "what is the faith that Christ is looking for when He comes to earth?" It has to be a faith that goes beyond belief in just truths or doctrines, but a faith in an entire way of life and state of being. This is the righteous, holy way that God Himself lives in and through us. He wants us to accept the whole way of life for Christians that is revealed in His Word, which says that we are to live by faith (John 17:3).

The *Be Real* philosophy is a way to examine ourselves to determine whether we are in the faith as Paul instructs us in 2 Corinthians 13:5. He tells us here to test ourselves to prove that Christ lives in us. We will not fail the test *if* we are truly trusting and depending on God to make the changes necessary to take on His nature as a way of life.

The *Be Real* Acronym is a ministry tool that seeks to stimulate and support the ongoing spiritually transforming work of the Holy Spirit in and through our personal lives, relationships, and ministries. This is so that we can progressively become more conformed to the image of Christ according to the will of God the Father. Will Christ Find *real* faith when He comes to earth?

Examine yourself. Test your faith and then answer with an astonishing ***yes***!

B -- Do you ***believe*** in God the Father, Son, and Holy Spirit?
E -- Are you ***experiencing*** power over your sins and yourself?
R -- Are you the ***righteousness*** of Christ Jesus?

E -- Are you Expecting ***eternal*** life?
A -- Have you ***accepted*** Christ as your Lord and Savior?
L -- Are you Living a life of ***love***?

It is a genuine faith walk that makes a *real* Christian. Not *rules* or *religion,* but ***relationship***!

The purpose of Be Real Fit™ is to get you to a place where you obey God in every area of your life because you love Him. He commands us to love and care for our temples, our bodies, because they belong to Him. We do that by sanctifying our Spirits in the Word, getting proper rest, exercising, and eating nutritious foods. We believe in God, we believe in good nutrition, and we believe in moderation.

God's promises are still in effect! God promised eternal life to those who accept Jesus and Follow Him, however, our earthly experiences can sometimes cause us to question our assurance of a true relationship with God. In 1 John, we see a congregation going through this very thing. The entire fifth chapter deals with the issue of whether or not all that know Christ are *real* Christians. Take a moment and read 1 John 5 and consider Paul's answer to this question. He reassures us that God does what He says He's going to do. Once you enter into God's Kingdom, you are in. It's done, it's over, you're in. Heaven is a given and eternal life is yours if you believe and continue to believe in Jesus Christ. *Be Real* for life!

Points to Ponder

Let's get real with our faith

1. What do you consider the most challenging part of accepting the *Be Real Faith* philosophy of examining ourselves to ensure our faith is *real.*

    ____

    ____

    ____

    ____

2. What are your fears about your beliefs? Why do you have them?

    ____

    ____

    ____

    ____

3. Consider your spiritual growth, how would you rate it? Do you feel intimidated or victorious by the standards of Christian living?

    ____

4. Can you identify a time in your life when you resisted God or the belief in Christ as God?

CHAPTER SIX

Be Real Fitness: Exercise with Him in Mind

Our philosophy of fitness is quite different from most others. We believe that in order to optimize your health, you should first optimize your mind and spirit. We understand that most believers do not have the time or the desire to spend hours in the gym; especially with work, family, church, and social schedules to contend with. Yet the bibles says, above all things we are to prosper and be in good health, even as our soul prospers (3 John1:2). How can our souls prosper if we are not feeding our bodies the nutrients it needs in order to perform at its best?

The body is the temple of the living God; our most prized possession, so why do we continue to feed it junk? Many do not look at the temptation of food as an attack from the devil, but it actually is! The fat demon is *real,* therefore we must Be *real* about our fitness; especially if we are going to withstand the attack of the enemy on our bodies and minds.

Be Real Fit™ has developed **Rhema**-*cises* with you in mind! **Rhema**-*cises* consists of various exercises that are used together according to your fitness level. They are designed to bring your body into its highest level of fitness so that you are able to look and feel your level best. How would you like to be able to exercise in the morning and still have the rest of your day to enjoy your friends and family? How would you like to turn your exercise program into a daily devotional designed to impact your life and improve your well-being?

Before we bring you **Rhema**-*cises*, we first have to look at the art and science of weight loss. This will answer the questions most of us have that keep us defeated. Questions like, "why does weight loss work for some people and not for others," or "why is it that some people lose weight on fad diets and others gain weight?" Many fail to launch into another diet and exercise program because of the past failures.

The first thing you are going to have to learn about the Be Real Fit™ philosophy is that we believe *all* people are capable of achieving their goals if they believe. Belief is the thing we must bring to the forefront of our minds if we are going to achieve any amount of success. Are you going to believe your past, or are you going to step out on faith. Faith says, I am going to look into what I am doing to see how I can do it a little better. This kind of knowledge deepens our awareness, and empowers us to ask the questions that can actually move us further in our goals.

For example, do you believe that you had the healthiest beverage possible this morning? If not, faith says I can change my beverage of choice to water and save 300 calories. Will walking actually cause me to lose weight, or am I just exercising for the sake of saying I did it? There are a lot of assumptions that overshadow our faith and keeps us on the roller coaster of yo-yo dieting, only to end up in a worse condition then when we started.

Let's look at weight and health from a different perspective to see if we can come up with a Rhema program that is designed just for you. The best way to lose weight is to approach it the way you approach everything else. How do you respond emotionally and psychologically to conflict, pain, frustration, and setbacks? If you can master your emotions and automatic responses, then you can master every other limitation and pattern that hinders your progress. Take the time to write your life's vision and imagine how it would be impacted based on your current health or weight status. Now write down your personal values and life's purpose to see how that plays a role in your everyday life choices. Together, we are going to co-create a fitness regimen that is going to help you reach your health, nutrition, fitness, and weight management goals.

Habits and mindsets can be broken, but first we must discover what you believe and how it is affecting your goals.

1. What do you believe about genetics?
2. What is your belief about hormones
3. How does environment play a role in your efforts?
4. What do you believe about calories?
5. How do you relate to food?

Now it's time to think and listen. Begin to list all of the other things that may affect or impact your health and wellness goals. Once you have the obstacles written down, begin to think about your actual exercise and weight loss goals and see if they are in proportion to the obstacles. If the obstacles out weigh the goals, stop and listen to something inspirational such as music or the spoken word. If your goals are bigger than the obstacles, remember your goals and do, watch, or listen to something that motivates you to continue. It may be possible that you have set out on your journey without the proper knowledge and tools to achieve your goals.

Now, let's put what we've just learned into practice. Considering how you handle things in your everyday life, your life and fitness goals, and how motivated you are, answer the following questions. Your answers will help us to create your fitness regime.

- On a scale of 1-10, how much do you believe you can achieve the fitness goal you have set for yourself?
- How badly do you want to achieve your goals?
- What do you think needs to be done in order to get you where you need to be?
- Who are the people who are going to partner with you to get you there?

Rhema-*cises* only require ten minutes in the morning and ten minutes in the evening, but must be done consistently on a daily basis. Long drawn out workouts are things of the past, and gym memberships are so unnecessary. You no longer need to spend hours on treadmills, elliptical machines, and exercise bikes; just pick ***five*** exercises and get a stopwatch. The routines are simple and results phenomenal.

You have everything you need right in your living room, and we are here to support you in your efforts. Our fitness coaches are all personal trainers and are experienced in helping clients reach their fitness goals. There is a workout for every fitness level and everyone can benefit from this one of a kind workout system.

Be Real Fit!™ Exercises

Horizontal Arm Swing:

1. Begin by standing tall with your feet shoulder width apart.
2. Holding your arms straight out to the side, then bring them forward and cross them over each other in one fluid motion.
3. Return to the starting position and repeat for the desired amount of time.

This exercise can be used to warm-up the upper body, take forward rotation out of shoulders, and release tension in the neck and shoulders.

High Knee Drill:

1. Stand at the foot of an agility ladder. If you do not have an agility ladder, simply stand in place.
2. Drive knee up towards chest and place that foot in first square or back on the ground.
3. Drive the other knee up and land in next square and so on down the ladder in a moderate to fast jog with minimal ground contact time. If you do not have an agility ladder, remain in place.

This exercise can be used to warm-up the lower body and release tension in the hips, low back, and shoulders.

Burpees:

1. From a standing position, jump as high as possible and land on your feet with your hands on the ground.
2. Kick your feet back (for a moment you will be in a push up position) and jump back up again as quickly as possible.
3. Repeat this exercise for the required duration.

This exercise boosts the heart rate, burns fat, and builds endurance. It also establishes a connection between the upper body and the lower body, and multiple planes of motion.

Standard Pushup:

1. Lie face down on the floor with hands palm down, fingers pointing straight ahead, and aligned at the nipple line.
2. Place hands slightly wider than shoulder width, and feet should be at hip width with toes on floor.
3. Start position: Extend the elbows and raise the body off the floor.

4. Lower your entire body (legs, hips, trunk, and head) four to eight inches from the floor.
5. Return to the start position by extending at the elbows and pushing the body up.
6. Remember to keep the head and trunk stabilized in a neutral position by isometrically contracting the abdominal and back muscles. Never fully lock out the elbows at the start position and avoid hyperextension of the low back.

This exercise can be used to build upper body and core strength.

Saggital Front Reach:
1. Start by standing with feet hip width apart. Hold a medicine ball or dumbbell at waist level.
2. Step forward two to three feet with the heel striking first and lean torso forward. With both hands, reach down towards the front foot so that finger tips touch the floor. ***Do not*** allow front knee to extend past the big toe as this may cause injury.
3. Pushing off front foot, return to start position. Continue with the same leg or alternate as prescribed.
4. Remember to keep head and back in a neutral position. Reaching forward should be performed at the hips and not the low back. Shoulders and hips should remain squared at all times.
5. Watch for proper knee alignment and remember not to let the front of the knee extend past the big toe or deviate laterally or medially. The back knee should not come in contact with floor.

This exercise can help build lower body strength especially in the hips and Gluteus Maximus (glutes).

Dumbbell Deadlift Row:
1. Begin by holding dumbbells at your side.
2. Squat down until the dumbbells almost touch the ground.
3. Proceed to stand up and stop when your legs are semi straight and your back is at a 45 degree angle.
4. Now, pull the dumbbells in towards your waist.
5. Return to the starting position and repeat as desired.

This exercise builds full body strength, especially in the glutes, lower back, upper back, and core.

Single Leg Plank Raise:

1. Start by forming a straight plank with your forearms and feet as the contact points on the ground.
2. Once the plank is formed raise one foot off the ground and then return to the starting position.
3. Repeat this movement for the desired repetitions alternating back and forth between your legs.

This exercise is great for building core and glute strength.

Lateral Step Up with Hop:
1. Stand to left side of box and place right foot on top of box.
2. Push off the box using the right leg only and explode vertically as high as possible. Drive the arms forward and up for maximum height.
3. Land with opposite foot onto box. Repeat with the other foot.
4. Repeat according to prescribed number of repetitions.

This exercise is great for burning fat and calories, boosting endurance, and improving balance and agility.

Quad Psoas Stretch:
1. Start by placing one knee on the balance disc with the foot on top of the stability ball.
2. Your other leg should be bent 90 degrees at the knee with your foot flat on the floor.
3. Slowly slide your foot on the floor forward and lean with your upper body towards the floor until a comfortable but moderate stretch is felt.
4. Return to the starting position and repeat or hold for desired amount of time if you would like.
5. Repeat with the other leg.

This exercise releases tension and helps to lengthen the hip flexors, inner thighs, glutes, and shoulders.

Downward Facing Dog:
1. Stand with feet hip width apart with your toes facing forward. Place the hands shoulder width apart and spread the fingers. Keep the tailbone lifted towards the sky and gently push down through the heels. Open the upper back by rotating the shoulder blades away from one another.
2. Keep the shoulders away from the ears and press down firmly through all fingers and thumbs. Spread the fingers push down through index and thumbs. Place more weight onto the feet than the hands.
3. Pull the navel towards the spine and lift the pelvic floor muscles. Drop

the ribcage towards the spine and lift the kneecaps up, then contract the quadricep muscles.
4. Maintain this pose for five to ten deep breaths.

This exercise releases tension and helps to lengthen the hamstrings, calves, abs, and upper back.

Dumbbell Squat:
1. Stand feet shoulder width apart with a 5 to 10 pound weight held on each shoulder.
2. Squat down until thighs are parallel to the floor, ***do not*** allow knees to extend past ankles.
3. Slowly return to start and repeat.

This exercise increases muscle strength, endurance, and balance hormones.

Dumbbell Lunge:
1. Hold a 5 to 10 pound dumbbell on each shoulder.
2. Take a 2 or 3 foot step forward, bending front knee to 90 degrees, make sure knee ***does not*** go over your ankle. Upper body should stay straight.
3. Slowly return to start and repeat on other side.
3. Triple arms dumbbell

This exercise increases muscle strength, endurance, and balance hormones.

Triple Arms Dumbbell:
1. Stand with feet shoulder width apart holding a 5 to 10 pound dumbbells with arms at your waist.
2. Lift weights toward chin, keeping hands close to body. Make sure not to arch back.
3. Return to start.

1. Place arm at your sides with 5 to 10 pound dumbbell in each hand.
2.. Keeping arms close to sides, curl one weight up, rotating wrist so palms face shoulders.
3.. Return to start, repeat on other side.

1. Holding 5 to 10 pound dumbells, stand with knees slightly bent and feet hip-width apart.

2. Bend slightly at the waist, extending arms back and lift.
3. Slowly drop arms and repeat.

Repeat the entire circuit. This exercise increases muscle strength, endurance, and balance hormones.

For optimum results, add 20 - 30 minutes of cardio exercise such as walking, jogging, or dancing two or three times a week.

Points to Ponder

Let's get Fit

Pick five different exercises from the previous page and list them below. Do three sets of 10, 12, and 15, each time adding intensity and weight while decreasing the amount of time it takes to do a round. Rest for 20 seconds and repeat before moving to the next move.

Rhema-*cises* for today

1. ______________________________

2. ______________________________

3. ______________________________

4. ______________________________

5. ______________________________

Each day, you will choose a scripture to meditate on during your **Rhema**-*cises* and throughout the day. You should also select inspirational music that will accompany the exercises you chose and get moving!

Rhema-*cise* Scripture for today

1. ____

CHAPTER SEVEN

Be Slim For Life

Let's talk about eating to *Be Slim,* and the role that food plays in our Be Real Fit™ goals. Snacking for many is the rate-limiting factor in getting those unwanted pounds off for good. Why is that? The reason is that unless you are able to get the same satisfaction that comes from eating from some other activity, you will always fall back into what you know and what is familiar to you. For many, food provides a sense of comfort and joy simply because our favorite foods are sometimes connected to an emotional or biological experience that stems from childhood. In this reactionary process, the pleasure far outweighs any vain desire to look good and feel better about one's self. It is imperative that we pinpoint what is happening with food in order to overcome this process.

What are the reasons you have failed in the past, and what is your relationship with food now? Think about what you have recently eaten and how it made you feel. The bible says to guard your heart and mind that you may not sin. The book of Ephesians talks about how we must put on the full armor of God. Part of this armor is the breastplate of righteousness; this is how we guard our hearts. The bible says in 1 John that if our hearts don't condemn us, we will have confidence before God. When guilt seeps in, our hearts should convict us, not condemn us.

To have a condemning heart means to have a heart of judgment. This type of heart knows its sin, but doesn't ask for and receive forgiveness for those sins. Rather than sabotaging and degrading oneself for a lack of discipline, allow the conviction to motivate you to do something different. The heart will always take you further than you want to go and test you beyond your personal limits. So rather than setting limitations and boundaries, we will become your accountability partner. Together we will create a skill set that will empower your mind, whether you are motivated to eat right or not.

You are going to create your own mantra and work it according to your own ability. A mantra is a sound, syllable, word, or group of words that is considered capable of "creating transformation." This is *your* language, *your* way, and it's going to propel you to reach *your* fitness goal because you are going to make it happen. Remember, the *Be Real* philosophy is based on what you believe, therefore, your mantra is in direct proportion to your ability. Here are a few examples.

1. I will plan my meals and have breakfast and dinner at home.

2. I will live the *Be Slim* way everyday except for Sunday when I will have one meal of choice.

3. I will eat only when I'm hungry, and stop when I'm full.

4. My cut off time for food is 7 PM daily and 2 PM for carbs.

5. Even If I do not feel like it, I am going to inspire myself to greatness everyday.

Now write your own mantra and take charge of your choices. It doesn't matter how big or how small. It may be as simple as, *I will drink water rather than soda* or *eat meals sitting rather than driving*. You take the wheel; no one is going to stop you from achieving the goals you set for yourself. This is extremely powerful and does not require much motivation. You believe in yourself and count on your word.

You are probably wondering what the *Be Slim* way of life is. *Be Slim* is an acronym for the foods we are to eat daily for optimum health and weight.

***Be Slim* For Life!**

B -- Beans and Berries: Most days, eat at lease a cup of beans and berries.

E -- Eggs: Eat eggs one to two times a week instead of meat.

S -- Salads, soups, stir fry, and steamed veggies: Steamed vegetables are the center of your meals. Fill up on raw, juiced, and cooked or steamed green vegetables. You can also include tomatoes, alfalfa and barley grass, broccoli, cabbage, celery, cucumber, dandelion, fresh cut green beans, garlic, leeks, onions, Rhubarb, Savoy cabbage, soy sprouts, spinach, wheat grass, zucchini, and red radish.

L -- Lean meats: Enjoy up to 4oz of lean meats to include fish such as flounder, sole, or tilapia three days a week. You can also eat nuts and seeds daily, up to 1oz or a handful.

I -- Include good fats: Consume good fats such as ground flaxseed, 1 tablespoon per meal, and small amounts of avocado or olive oil.

M -- Monitor carbs: Include whole grain carbs include starchy vegetables, corn, brown rice, carrots, and small potatoes.

A typical *Be Slim* day can consist of the following meals:

Early Morning: Fruit or vegetable juices
Breakfast: Whole grain cereal or bagel with low fat cream cheeses
Midday: Fruit or vegetable juices
Lunch: Beans, lean meat or eggs, or nuts with salad greens and olive oil
Dinner: Two cooked greens, optional 4oz meat or one cup of whole grains or starchy vegetables with good fat

After two or three weeks of detox, your *Be Slim* day will look slightly different. Here is an example of post detox *Be Slim* meals.

Early Morning	Fruit
Breakfast	One or two eggs, whole grain English muffin or bagel, 1 teaspoon of margarine or cream cheese or 1 cup of protein enriched cereal with 2/3 cups of milk
Lunch	3 ounces of deli meat, 1/4 cup beans, 2 tablespoons low-fat cheese, 3 cups mixed salad, 2 tablespoons light dressing, 6 triscuits or 1 can of tuna, 2 tablespoons celery, 1 tablespoons of light mayo, 1 whole wheat pita or bread, 1/2 cup veggies, 2 tablespoons of light dressing
Dinner	4oz chicken breast, 1 tablespoon Teriyaki sauce, 1/2 cup of brown rice, 1 teaspoon of nuts, 1 cup of steamed vegetables or 3oz of cooked shrimp or lean beef, 1/4 cup of shredded or 1 slice of fat free cheese, 3 cups mixed baby spinach, 2 tablespoons of light dressing or condiments, 1 whole wheat dinner roll with 1 teaspoon of margarine.
Snack	4oz greek plain yogurt, 1 hard boiled egg or 1 stick of string cheese, with 1 cup of berries or citrus fruit with 3 crackers or few almonds

Because I'm healthy, I'm eating healthy!

This is our way of eating to maintain a healthy body fat percentage and weight range. We do not believe in starving ourselves, nor do we believe in eating beyond our natural capacity to feel full. Look at your meals from this perspective, when you are driving your car, what is it that makes it go and keeps it going? Fuel! That's exactly what protein is for your body. It fuels your muscles and is what keeps it going. Therefore at every meal there should be a small amount of protein, or you risk running out of fuel and wasting precious muscle.

In that same car, what keeps the engine from overheating and makes the car run smoothly? That's right, the oil! That's what good fats do for the body. They lubricate the cell membranes and keep your brain functioning properly.

When the car is not properly running, what does it usually need? You got it, a tune-up or a bit of fine-tuning. That's what carbs do for the body. They are only minimally needed because they are not the fuel or the water, which is vital in order for the car to run. A car can go a very long time without a tune-up, just like the body can go without carbs. However, eventually the body runs out of energy and will require unrefined, high quality sources of energy that come from high fibrous grains to psychologically feel good. How much you need is based on your own wisdom and intuition. However, whole grains beyond three servings will go to the hips and waistline if not burned off through physical activity.

High processed foods never work for anyone at anytime. There is a bigger problem than just eating the right kinds of food, and the *Be Slim* plan addresses the hormonal effect of food. It is a lie to say, *a calorie is a calorie*, or *calorie in, calorie out* is the way to lose weight. All calories do not act the same way within the body. The hormonal effect makes all the difference in what a calorie does.

If a calorie comes from sugar, insulin is going to be released from the pancreas, which goes into the bloodstream to remove the sugar. If we are active and metabolic syndrome has not set in, then the sugar would be used for energy as the insulin carries it into all the muscle's cells. Lack of sleep, inactivity, stress, and processed foods cause high levels of cortisol, which makes this process of insulin moving sugar into the bloodstream impossible. The muscles and fat cells become resistant to the effects of insulin. If it continues, the pancreas cannot do its job and the sugar levels increase because the insulin is not able to move sugar into the bloodstream. The result is that you become a diabetic and obese.

So where are you going to start? Do not attempt to completely change your lifestyle all at once or go about this on your own. Get additional help on your journey from one of our coaches or fitness professionals. We can help you get past your mental block and get you to a place where healthy choices are part of your daily life.

You may be wondering what the best vegetables are for optimum health? It's as simple as knowing the colors of the rainbow, and how each one benefits your health and overall nutrition.

Green Foods: Green foods such as broccoli, kale, cabbage, and spinach are good for the circulatory system.

Orange Foods: Orange foods such as carrot, pumpkin, and apricots help to prevent cancer by repairing the DNA and improve eye sight.

***Red Foods*:** Red foods such as tomatoes, watermelon, and red cabbage reduce sun damage to the skin.

Green/Yellow Foods: Green/Yellow foods such as yellow corn, avocado, and collard greens reduce the risk of developing cataracts and macular degeneration. They also reduce the risk of osteoporosis.

Orange/Yellow Foods: Orange/Yellow foods such as pineapple, tangerine, and papaya improve the health of the mucus membrane and connective tissue, and prevent heart disease by improving circulation and preventing inflammation.

White/Green Foods: White/Green foods such as onions, pears, and celery reduce the effects of potentially toxic, high fat meats and help to keep joint fluids healthy.

Red/Purple/Blue Foods: Foods such as blackberries, strawberries, and red apples protect against heart disease by improving circulation and preventing blood clots.

**For optimum results, choose two vegetables per meal*

The use of supplements is usually a controversial topic, however, the *Be Slim* philosophy is that they are necessary for optimum health. Multivitamins, Vitamin D, and Omega 3 fatty acids are necessary to increase the likelihood of the body being nourished and to prevent chronic disease such as diabetes, hypertension, cancer risk, rheumatoid arthritis, and multiple sclerosis.

The overall philosophy of the *Be Slim* way of life is to eat for nourishment and optimum health. We are living in an age of compulsive eating that creates sickly individuals whose lifestyles require the use of pharmaceuticals to manage their health. I am a Pharmacist by profession, and I know first hand that medication does not cure or prevent disease. The truth is, food can improve your health and prevent disease from occurring in the first place.

The *Be Slim* plan is a seven week optimum eating program that includes recipes and scriptures to transform your life and body. This plan requires a no compromise commitment and attitude, but the results will be simply remarkable. You will feel better, sleep better, and look better. This seven week intensive program is designed to rid food addicts of compulsion, and get them on the road to recovery and wellness.

Points to Ponder

Let's get Slim

1. Since starting this book, what have you discovered about yourself and how you relate to food?

____

____

____

____

2. What are you committed to doing differently to support your decision to live the *Be Slim* way everyday?

____

____

____

____

CHAPTER EIGHT

Be Real Fellowship: Relationships Matter

The first phase of a relationship is fellowship with our creator. Fellowship involves having conversations with Him about the desires and plans of His heart, not ours. The bible says in James 4:8, *Draw near to God and He will draw near to you.* Fellowship with God also involves worshiping Him. How is it that many people expect to receive from God, yet they do not have a relationship with or worship Him? Can we expect to receive the promises of God without being in fellowship with Him? The gift of salvation is all we need to be in right relationship with God, yet many people today, including those in the church, want God to fix the problems they have without coming into agreement or relationship with Him and His Word.

People of the world are no longer satisfied with money, cars, and houses; they are now looking for more personal satisfaction. Jesus said in John 3:3, "I tell you the truth, no one can see the Kingdom of God unless He is born again." Having a relationship with God, ourselves, and others that is healthy requires showing sacrificial love. The reason that many people do not have faithful, godly relationships is because of the unrealistic expectations we place upon each other. The bible says that trials and suffering are common to every human being, including believers, but they should bring us closer together and make us stronger. God promises to provide strength to see us through and an eternal hope that makes the temporary suffering we experience in relationships bearable. But we must have a realistic view of our expectations for each relationship, including spiritual ones.

Within us lives the power of the Holy Spirit, therefore we can have extraordinary and meaningful relationships with one another without the pressures of lust, anger, rage, and covetousness. Many people are hurt, but that is not an excuse not to give a warm smile, hug, or kind gesture. It can literally change someone's life and have a lasting impact on someone whose spirit is low and needs to be lifted.

Positive thinking plays a role in how we perceive one another in relationships. If you think positively, positive things will happen. Negative thoughts lead to negative responses. The goal of every believer should be, to glorify God in our relationships. We can achieve this by treating the cares of the world as if they are temporal. Revelation 21:3-4 says, *And I heard a great voice out of heaven saying, Behold, the tabernacle of God is with men, and he will dwell with them, and they shall be his people, and God Himself shall be with them, and be their*

God. And God shall wipe away all tears from their eyes, and there shall be no more death, sorrow, nor crying, neither shall there be any more pain for the former things are passed away.

The fullness of God's care will be experienced in the new heaven and new earth. This includes wiping all tears and removing all pain from our earthly opposition. All the things we are experiencing now are passing away, and God is sitting on the throne making all things new. The new creation will not only be fixed up old bodies, but we will have new glorious bodies if we overcome. Therefore, as much as we wish to be completely free in our relationships now, the truth is that we are not and will not be completely free until the day Christ returns. As difficult as it may appear at times, we can have peace and harmony in our present relationships if we learn to enjoy the finite capabilities we have right now. In the new bodies, our relationships will be deepened and we all will be pure and prepared to be a bride.

Christians have sinned and done some abominable things, yet we all have been forgiven because of the Lamb of God. We should then treat each other as one who has been forgiven and redeemed. We should separate the sin of a person from the person so that we are able to love them past where they are. In the new heaven, there will be no sin, no rejection, or casting out. Every threat will be removed and the gate will be constantly opened. Can we do that with our hearts now? Of course we can, but only by the power of the Holy Spirit! By focusing only on that which glorifies God and is good for His people, we can experience the wonderful life on earth that Christ did with his friends and disciples.

A willingness to accept and allow personal change is the pathway to wellness in our relationships. We must start with our relationship with God, ourselves, and then one another. We must also consider our faith. We can all give brotherly love and not live in constant strife and conflict. This leads to malice and eventually disease.

BE REAL FIT

Program Guide: A Pathway to Wellness through
FAITH, FITNESS AND FELLOWSHIP

This program is for people who are tired of being defeated in mind, body, spirit, and soul and who would like to be encouraged and empowered to reach optimum health and wellness. The Be Real Fit™ wellness lifestyle is designed to give you optimum health and weight through powerful interactive coaching sessions and *Be Real* Talks. We have gathered the best team of professionals to provide you with an individualized plan that moves you through the seven week, proven pathway to wellness.

Here is what you can expect from the Be Real Fit™ coaching program!

1. **Learn to prepare and enjoy food for optimum health and wellness.** Calories are not created equal. What you eat is just as important as how much you eat. Get connected with your inner wellness and let it lead you to making better choices. *Be Slim* nutritionist have designed meal plans that are guaranteed to maximize your results. You can expect to:
   - Optimize weight loss and break through plateaus
   - Release toxins from your cells that are draining your energy and altering your hormones
   - Enjoy eating healthy food without feeling deprived
   - Not yield to cravings and rid yourself of emotional eating for good
   - Eat to balance hormones that affect your weight, sleep quality, energy, and metabolism
2. **Let's Rhema-*cise*! Exercises designed with you in mind.** If you hate exercising, it's not because you weren't meant to do it. You just haven't found a workout tailor made for you. **Rhema-***cise* is the type of exercise that you will actually stick to because

it's perfectly matched with your personality. Wherever you are and whatever you are doing, there is always time to **Rhema**-*cise*. During the *Be Slim* seven week intensive program, you will:

- Learn how to find your Rhema workout
- Customize your fitness plan with simple, but effective exercises that tone, lift, and slim
- Learn how exercise can be done anytime and anywhere.

3. **Be ye transformed by the renewal of your mind.** Transformation can only truly take place when you finally confirm with yourself that you are beautifully, fearfully, and wonderfully made. You will learn to love the body you're in while being empowered to move into the body you so desire. No more excuses, just commitment.
4. **Accept what is and change what isn't.** Your surroundings often mirror what's going on inside your body. Stress, clutter, and excess can all lead to a false sense of being overwhelmed. Let's face it, surroundings that are tailored to our preference can really help us reach our weight loss goals. Look around and lets get rid of all that does not belong. Replace it with what fits our *now*.
6. **Nourish and foster healthy relationships.** Relationships are important, and play a vital role in our overall well-being. Family, friends, coworkers, and others can all contribute to or hinder your *Be Slim/Be Real Fit*™ goals. Life is better with positive relationships. There are no bad people, just bad relationships. Lets heal and be set free.
7. **Faith built to last.** Where is your faith? In order to have lasting results, there must be a spiritual foundation that can withstand the test of time. No more being spiritual rookies; let's use the Word of God to be what we were created to be, and use our faith to reach our goals.
8. **Be Real Fit™ for Life.** Walk into your wellness destiny and learn how to keep the weight off for the rest of your life. Time to celebrate your accomplishment, hard work, and dedication.

CHAPTER NINE

What Does the Word Say

Maybe you are struggling with making healthy choices and sticking to the commitment that you have made to change your lifestyle. God has promised you in his word that He will be with you, even until the end of the world (Matthew 28:20). He will be with you as you make the choice to eat a healthy, balanced meal, as well as when you make the decision to exercise and move your body. Always remember that God is faithful to keep His promises.

The Lord is faithful to all His promises and loving toward all He has made. The Lord upholds all those who fall and lifts up all who are bowed down.

Psalm 145:13-14

It's easy to give in to snack cravings and choose unhealthy options for certain meals. Let's face it, chocolate is yummy and hamburgers are delicious, but with God all things are possible; even resisting cravings and the urge to eat unhealthy foods.

Walk in the Spirit, and you shall not fulfill the lust of the flesh. For the flesh lusts against the Spirit and the Spirit against the flesh; and these are contrary to one another, so that you do not do the things that you wish. But if you are led by the Spirit, you are not under the law. Now the works of the flesh are evident, which are: adultery, fornication, uncleanness, lewdness, idolatry, sorcery, hatred, contentions, jealousies, outbursts of wrath, selfish ambitions, dissensions, heresies, envy, murders, drunkenness, revelries, and the like; of which I tell you beforehand, just as I also told you in time past, that those who practice such things will not inherit the kingdom of God.

Galatians 5:16-21

Some of you may have recently realized that giving in to gluttony and overindulgence is a sin. As with any other sin, ask God for forgiveness and work towards making better food choices. If we ask for forgiveness, God is faithful and just to forgive us for our sin.

If we confess our sins, he is faithful and just and will forgive us our sins and purify us from all unrighteousness.

1 John 1:9

Are you feeling as if you are different from others around you? Well here's the truth. You are! The bible identifies Christians as a peculiar people. We are set apart from the world and should be confident in our uniqueness. Therefore we should find comfort in the Word of God rather than food and inappropriate relationships as the world does.

Do not love the world or the things in the world. If anyone loves the world, the love of the Father is not in him. For all that is in the world -- the lust of the flesh, the lust of the eyes, and the pride of life -- is not of the Father but is of the world. And the world is passing away, and the lust of it; but he who does the will of God abides forever.
1 John 2:15

Write down your own faith, fitness, and fellowship confession of where you are and where you want to be. Allow the Lord to heal, deliver, and set you free!

About the Author

Loranda "Victorious" Thomas, Rph is a virtuous woman of God who has a heart and love for God's people. She is married to Pastor Hermie Thomas, Jr and her greatest joy is her two children Judah 13, and Royal 12.

She is currently attending Fuller Theological Seminary in Houston, Texas where she is pursuing a Master of Arts in Theology and Ministry. As Co-Founder of Kingdom Living Center, her life long dream of serving alongside her husband in ministry is finally a reality.

As Chief Pharmacist of the City of Houston's Health Department and as a Certified Professional Coach, Loranda has helped hundreds of men and women successfully reach their health and wellness goals. As a new Author, Loranda hopes her book, *Be Real Fit: A Spiritual Pathway to Victorious Living,* will serve as a guide to those wanting to be fit; mind, body, spirit and soul.

PraiseMoves™ were developed by Laurette Willis as the Christian alternative to yoga. For more information, visit http://praisemoves.com/.

The food colors used for Be Real Fit! Program are courtesy of the Rainbow Food Chart.

Rhema-*cises* use various exercises that use your own body weight to promote weight loss. For an example of exercises included in **Rhema**-*cises*, visit http://www.freeworkoutsguide.com/.

Made in United States
North Haven, CT
04 November 2026

21765278R00051